The A
Medicine Made Easy

What You Need to Know about Great Ways in Treating Different Medical Condition

By: Adam Potts

9781680322286

Publishers Notes
Disclaimer – Speedy Publishing LLC

This publication is intended to provide helpful and informative material. It is not intended to diagnose, treat, cure, or prevent any health problem or condition, nor is intended to replace the advice of a physician. No action should be taken solely on the contents of this book. Always consult your physician or qualified health-care professional on any matters regarding your health and before adopting any suggestions in this book or drawing inferences from it.

The author and publisher specifically disclaim all responsibility for any liability, loss or risk, personal or otherwise, which is incurred as a consequence, directly or indirectly, from the use or application of any contents of this book.

Any and all product names referenced within this book are the trademarks of their respective owners. None of these owners have sponsored, authorized, endorsed, or approved this book.

Always read all information provided by the manufacturers' product labels before using their products. The author and publisher are not responsible for claims made by manufacturers.

This book was originally printed before 2014. This is an adapted reprint by Speedy Publishing LLC with newly updated content designed to help readers with much more accurate and timely information and data.

Speedy Publishing LLC

40 E Main Street, Newark, Delaware, 19711

Contact Us: 1-888-248-4521

Website: http://www.speedypublishing.co

REPRINTED Paperback Edition: ISBN: 9781680322286

Manufactured in the United States of America

Dedication

I dedicate this book to my late mother, Natalia. Thank you for your unconditional love and support.

Table of Contents

Publishers Notes 2

Dedication 3

Table of Contents 4

Chapter 1- Introduction to Alternative Medicine 5

Chapter 2- The Truth About Alternative Medicine 13

Chapter 3- Know Your Different Options in Alternative Medicine 24

Chapter 4- The Attributes of Herbs as Alternative Medicine 38

Chapter 5- Take Alternative Medicine for Anxiety, Depression and Cancer 43

Chapter 6- Alternative Medicine Affects Your Overall Wellness 49

Chapter 7- Herbal Teas Recipes as Alternative Medicine 56

About The Author 91

Chapter 1 - Introduction to Alternative Medicine

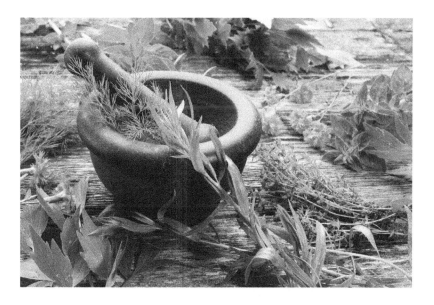

Traditionally, the first response for Americans to any type of medical issue is conventional medicine. There is, however, another option. Alternative medicine is sometimes considered the oldest medicine in the world.

Alternative medicine envelops the concept of seeking out non-traditional ways to deal with day-to-day health issues. This type of medicine looks beyond taking medication.

People look to use alternative medicine for two main reasons. The first is because of the idea that taking medications can potentially lead to unhealthy results such as dependencies and side effects. The second is because of the natural curiosity of man to find better methods to heal.

Alternative medicine encompasses many different therapies, such as hypnosis, color therapy, yoga, meditation, herbal remedies, vitamin therapy, and many more.

The Art of Alternative Medicine Made Easy

The main focus of alternative medicine is that life is a combination of parts that includes more than the treatment of disease. There is a definite focus on living life well, happily, and with purpose. It is believed that this is an essential part of healthy living.

This guide will explore the many different components of alternative medicine, and how it can help you. Consider using the ideas captured here next time you feel ill to begin feeling better naturally.

Treatments Beyond Conventional

When most people get sick, they look to conventional methods of medical treatment for relief and healing. There are alternative methods to treatment that are becoming increasingly popular.

What treatments are considered "conventional?" Prescription medication, traditional surgery, and computerized scientific testing are three examples of conventional medicine. Most physicians support conventional medicine in their practices, so when seeing a doctor, it is highly likely you will be advised to follow conventional medical advice.

The decision to use conventional medicine should be made by the patient and doctor on a case by case basis. An alteration to the type of treatment is sometimes all that is needed to feel better.

Alternative treatments include:

- Herbal remedies

- Massage

- Meditation

- Acupuncture

- Many more!

Patients will often find themselves turning to alternative methods of treatment when conventional methods are ineffective or a medical problem has been deemed untreatable. Alternative treatments are designed to not only aid in pain relief, but also reduce stress and tension that can worsen chronic pain.

Alternative methods of treatment focus on the whole person; body and soul. Convention methods strictly focus on the physical problems alone. For alternative methods to be effective, the patient must be motivated and believe in the alternative treatment's ability to work.

Of course, any serious, life-threatening health problem should blend conventional and alternative methods for a comprehensive approach. Be sure to consult with your doctor to avoid complications. If planned well, you can take advantage of best of both types of medicine for a life that is comfortable and enjoyable.

Alternative Medicine History & Theory

Thousands of years ago, all medicine was "alternative medicine." Before modern science, healers would consider the full picture - emotional, physical, and spiritual – before healing a sick person.

This is one of the main differences between modern conventional medicine and alternative medicine. Alternative medicine does not look for the instant cure for the physical problem, rather is looks more at a long-term solution that includes the whole self.

The Art of Alternative Medicine Made Easy

Just a few centuries ago in Europe there were two types of healers; folk healers that used old tried-and-true methods, and professional physicians. The lower classes did not have the money to pay for the professional physicians, but they used the folk healers and it worked.

In North America, philosophy and religion were often used to help folk healers provide holistic treatments.

The conventional medicine that we have today has evolved from the days of folk healers and alternative medicine. Many conventional physician support different types of holistic treatments in the overall wellness plan for their patients. The reason that alternative medicine has stood the test of time is because it works!

Ancient Chinese Medicine

Traditional Chinese medicine (TCM) includes acupuncture, Qigong, herbal treatments, deep massage, and more. More than 25% of the world's population practices TCM.

Several reputable groups, such as the World Health Organization and the National Institute of Health, find traditional Chinese medicine to be a viable alternative to contemporary medicine.

Many parts of TCM began well over 3,000 years ago in China. The focus of TCM is Qi (pronounced "Chee"), which is the body's energy that connects it to the world around us. It is believed that all disorders and bodily problems are caused by the misalignment of Qi. Acupuncture is one of the most widely recognized methods of bringing the Qi into alignment.

Herbal remedies are popular in traditional Chinese medicine. They are used to relax and calm the patient's emotions to avoid depression, and provide a more positive outlook on the illness. This helps tremendously in the healing process. Ginseng and herbal green tea are the most popular herbal remedies in China.

Exercise, mainly Qigong (pronounce "Chee Kung"), is also an important part of traditional Chinese medicine. Qigong involves posture, meditation, and slow, calculated body movements.

Tibetan Medicine

Tibetan Medicine is almost solely based on herbal remedies, and has been around for over 2,500 years. It is called "gSoba Rig-pa". Tibetans mostly live in India because they have been in exile since the late 1950's. They practice Tibetan Buddhism.

There is a Tibetan Medical Institute in Northern India, where doctors studying Tibetan medicine attend for 7 years before earning a degree.

The underlying belief in Tibetan medicine is that all illnesses are caused by poisonous thinking which include dread, denial, and want. This concept ties to the principles of Buddhist philosophy.

The three poisonous thoughts are believed to be caused by poor diet, inappropriate behavior, and the imbalance of time and season. This concept is more complicated than this, but this simplification will give a general sense of it.

Cures are linked to all systems of the body working together. The elimination of sweat, feces and urine contributes to this harmony.

The Art of Alternative Medicine Made Easy

Similar to the Chinese "Qi", the Tibetans have the Rlung, which is the overall life force that connects us to the universe. Rlung has five types:

1. Centered in the brain. Life grasping – controls breathing, intellect, sneezing and swallowing.

2. Centered in the chest. Upward moving – controls verbal ability and stamina.

3. Centered in the heart. All pervading – controls all movement like that of the orifices of the body and walking.

4. Centered in the stomach. Fire accompanying – controls digestion and metabolism.

5. Centered in the rectum. Downward cleansing – controls everything that is expelled from the body, such as babies, menstrual blood or semen.

Tibetan medicine usually handles sickness diagnosis by analysis of the tongue and urine. The spiritual element is also at play in Tibetan medicine, with much attention spent focusing on the type and temperament of spirits in the body.

American Indian Medicine (aka Native American Medicine)

North American Indian tribes have been practicing medicine for what some claim to be over 40,000 years. The medical information and techniques are handed down from generation to generation; ensure the longevity of the practice.

Some remedies are tribe-specific, although all tribal medicine is called Native American Medicine, collectively. Native Americans believe that man is one with nature and that the elements provide strength and can cure disease.

It is fascinating to note that at the same time that Native American medicine was being practiced in North America, Traditional Chinese Medicine was being practiced a half a world away. Ayurveda (medicine practiced in India), was also practiced at this time, and will be covered next.

All of these traditional medical practices are based on the same fundamental belief that a person's lifestyle and environment should be taken into consideration before choosing a treatment path. There are subtle differences between the practices that are specific to the region.

Native American medicine recognizes a purification procedure involving herbal smoke before and after treatment. Treatments include the use of sage and cedar smoke to repel negative energy. Negative energy is considered the pain released by someone who is ill, or the pain that the healer takes on themselves from their patients. Therapeutic touch is used. Singing, chanting, drums and rattles accompany the healing during the session.

Ayurvedic Medicine

Ayurvedic Medicine is practiced in India, and focuses on natural healing. Practitioners believe that it is important for the body to be balanced, and all medicines are based on vegetables and minerals, with the active ingredients from plant alkaloids.

In Ayurvedic Medicine there is the belief that there are three elements in the body, called Kapha, Pitta, and Vata, that cause disease.

1. Kapha: This energy is caused by the lack of stabilizing the balance in the body. These are commonly called viruses by Westerners.

2. Pitta: This energy supports vision, temperature, hunger, thirst, intelligence, and happiness. When out of alignment, the outcomes include weight fluctuation, dehydration, depression, digestive issues, and apathy.

3. Vata: This energy keeps the overall balance between the earth, sky and world around us in check with ourselves. If it falls out of balance, sickness is invited in.

Disease is called Vyaadhi, and it is treated by focusing on the imbalance of elements.

Chapter 2 - The Truth About Alternative Medicine

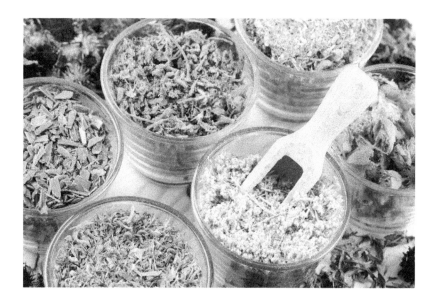

Mind and body are easily defined, but what is the "spirit" of you? The spirit, or soul, can be considered the part of you that is spiritually passionate. What makes you passionate? Here are a few ideas that can help you decide:

1. Look forward to something that you can anticipate.

2. Create a happy place where you can go when you meditate.

3. Reminisce about your successes.

4. Find something that relieves your stress and do it.

5. Explore your future goals – not money related.

The Art of Alternative Medicine Made Easy

Kama-Sutra

The Kama-Sutra is ancient text about sexual health that was written sometime between the 1st and 6th century in India. There are 35 chapters that cover everything from how to find a wife, to how to perform in bed, to how to make yourself attractive to others.

Sections of the book cover the relationship between diet and sexual wellbeing. Wholesome, nutritious foods are specifically referenced. Histamines are recommended, through food, for increased sexual pleasure.

Breathing techniques are stressed. This helps ease stress and improves overall sexual health.

Feng Shui

Feng Shui is the concept of bring nature and natural patterns and surroundings into our homes and everyday lives. This will bring harmony and peaceful alignment with the world.

Feng Shui brings together all of the elements. Fire, earth, air, and water, and the additional "metal", are represented inside the home by the selection of lighting, scents, sounds, and the placement of furniture and fixtures.

The underlying concept is that the qi, or life force, must be able to move freely in a room. Therefore, the location of furniture, for example, is important.

Chiropractics

Chiropractics are an alternative medicinal practice that is now considered conventional. The main theory behind chiropractics is that the vertebrate of the spine is not in alignment. It is believed that this misalignment causes many diseases and disorders throughout the body.

Chiropractors use pressure to realign and adjust the spine. Most chiropractors also look at the whole picture – stress, lifestyle choices, and overall health – when recommending treatment.

Chiropractors have been known to heal a wide range of medical problems through their work on patient's backs. Asthma, migraines, arthritis and more issues can all be positively impacted.

This treatment is safe and usually inexpensive. It is non-evasive. Going to a chiropractor will certainly require regular visits because your issues will not be fully treated in just one session.

Biofeedback

Biofeedback is a tool used to gauge internal function, then determine treatment, and then gauge if treatment is working properly. Similar to a thermometer or scale to measure the body weight or if there is a fever, biofeedback is garnered through tools.

The body function that it is measuring is activity that one cannot voluntarily control, such as blood pressure and brain wavelengths.

The main recommendation in alternative health for biofeedback is usually relaxation. This reduces the heart rate, calms the brain, and greatly impacts the affected parts of the body.

The Art of Alternative Medicine Made Easy
Using Alternative Medicine in Children

Sometimes conventional treatments are not an option for children. One example of when alternative medicines are a viable option for children is when they refuse to take their over-the-counter medication. They might be more willing to take an herbal remedy because it is something different.

Consider discussing with your conventional doctor these supplementary treatments for children:

• Acupuncture

The needles release endorphins to the brain which can help kids with asthma, and reduce other pains.

• Hypnosis

This technique might give a child more discipline regarding the regular administration of their conventional medication.

• Relaxation techniques and massage

This can help kids with asthma deal with constricting airways. Massage can help relax the stress surround asthma as well. Breathing techniques can help kids feel in control of their breathing. Kids with more serious diseases such as diabetes and cancer can use the relaxing benefits of massage to relieve stress and help maintain a positive outlook.

Always do plenty of research and consult with your child's doctor before beginning any alternative medical techniques.

Gender-Specific Alternative Medicine

Men and women each have their own medical needs specific to their gender. It is wise to consider what areas of alternative medicine are best geared for your gender.

For women, issues related to menstruation – such as regular menstruation and PMS are always hot topics. For these issues, women have the following homeopathic options:

- Acupuncture

- Chinese medicinal herbs & herbal teas

- Osteopathy

- Crystal therapy

- Yoga

- Hypnosis

For men, issues around prostate health and overall wellbeing can involve an alternative approach. Men have these choices:

- Yoga

- Acupuncture

- Herbal treatments

Men and women both need to care for their health. A proactive, homeopathic approach will ensure a happy, healthy life.

The Art of Alternative Medicine Made Easy
Homeopathic Weight Loss

There are alternative techniques that can be used in the fight to lose unwanted pounds. Of course, just like in conventional medicine, there is no magic pill.

However, the standard "eat well, be more active" technique of losing weight can be enhanced with alternative medicine.

First, you can consider yoga. This exercise is slow and calculated, but the results can be dramatic. When practices wholeheartedly and regularly, you can gain muscle and lose fat.

Acupuncture can reduce food cravings that are sabotaging your weight loss efforts. Teas can help curb cravings as well as detoxify the body.

Follow these tips to lose weight with alternative medicine:

1. Use a juicer to drink your fruits and vegetables.

2. Add Omega-3 to your beverages.

3. Visit a homeopathic doctor for a nutritional evaluation.

4. Contact an herbalist for recommendations on alternative teas.

5. Consider taking bovine or shark cartilage.

6. Hypnosis can be used for behavioral modification.

Alternative Medicine and Cancer

People with cancer often look for viable options that they can use to fight this disease. Unfortunately, there is no cure for cancer. Conventional treatments are the most aggressive, and while alternative and conventional medicine should work together to provide a comprehensive medical experience, at this time they do not.

You can use alternative medicine to supplement your conventional cancer treatments. Here are some of the best complementary alternative treatments:

1. Acupuncture: Helps with nausea, tiredness, pain, headaches.

2. Herbal remedies: Ginger, for one, is helpful in dealing with nausea and vomiting caused by chemotherapy.

3. Hyperbaric oxygen therapy is currently being studies as a complementary treatment for radiation therapy.

4. Massage helps relieve fatigue.

One of the biggest benefits of complimentary treatments is that the sick person can take control over their situation and treatment, even if just in a small way. This helps the patient's chances for survival and improves the quality of life.

As with any medical treatment, consult with your doctor before self-treating. Dangerous and counterproductive side effects can result if treatment is not cohesively planned.

The Art of Alternative Medicine Made Easy
What Happens in an Alternative Treatment Session?

First and foremost, it is essential to pick the right practitioner for you. When selecting your perfect practitioner, be sure to review their credentials because there are many fraudulent practitioners in the alternative medical world.

Follow these tips to find the perfect practitioner:

1. Search the phone book and online for local professionals. Select a local group of practitioners.

2. Research this group of practitioners to find out their experience, education, style, and anything else you can about them.

3. Find out what organizations they are affiliated with. The more trade groups, the better.

4. Contact them to ask what specific experience they have with your type of situation.

5. Ask what the treatment process is for your given situation.

The focus of an alternative medicine session is different then what occurs in a conventitional medical session. Here, the practitioner will want to learn about you as a whole person, not just the specific area of injury or concern.

How to Become an Alternative Medical Practitioner

Are you thinking about becoming an alternative medical practitioner? The profession is rewarding and interesting, and provides you with the opportunity to help people. By providing an alternative medicine service, you will be making a difference in the world.

First, you will need to determine which type of alternative medicine you want to practice. Alternative medicine is broken down into seven categories:

1. Dioelectricmagnetic applications

2. Diet

3. Nutrition

4. Lifestyle changes

5. Herbal medicine

6. Manual healing

7. Biological treatments

To become a professional alternative medicine practitioner, you will need to successfully complete an accredited program at a registered school. There are many schools that specialize in one area or another of alternative medicine.

Schooling is intensive, and a good program will include years of study and practice, as well as an internship experience.

Once you have completed school and practicum work you will be able to practice your field of study on your own.

The Art of Alternative Medicine Made Easy
Paying for Alternative Medicine

Prices for alternative treatments vary. Most treatments are not covered by insurance, so it is important to discuss actual costs prior to rendering services from a practitioner.

The first step in finding out how to pay for treatment is to call your insurance company to see if they will cover your treatment session. If they do cover, find out the specifics. How many sessions? Is there a specific type of treatment that is only covered?

When you meet your practitioner, one of the first questions to ask is if they accept your type of insurance. If you are not using insurance, you will need to work out alternative payment.

In North America, alternative medicine has experienced an increase in popularity in recent years. Of course, there is controversy surrounding the two big types of medicine; conventional and traditional.

With all of the wonderful benefits of alternative medicine, there are some risks associated with it. The follow risks should be considered before using alternative medicine:

1. Unsafe, ineffective, untested substances

2. Listening to exaggerated claims of safety by some unscrupulous businesses

3. Forgoing conventional treatments for serious illnesses to use an alternative treatment.

4. Not disclosing the simultaneous use of both conventional and alternative treatments, possibly creating a negative health situation

It is important to recognize possible risks in alternative medicine. As with anything, if a therapy, product or substance sound like it is too good to be true – then it probably is!

Always research the therapy or substance, as well as any practitioners that you are thinking about using. Check credentials and references, if possible. Because much of the alternative medicine world is unregulated, there are frauds out there that you will need to be weary of.

If you are careful about what you put in your body, and the types of external therapy you solicit, you can make educated choices that will benefit your health greatly.

The best approach is a strategically planned approach that you create and discuss with your doctor. If you are not comfortable talking with your conventional medical doctor about supplementing with alternative medicine treatments, then find one that is open minded about this type of treatment. You will be happy you did.

Only once you have research all the different alternative treatments from around the world will you have a full understanding about what options are actually out there. The internet is an excellent place to begin your research journey.

Chapter 3 - Know Your Different Options in Alternative Medicine

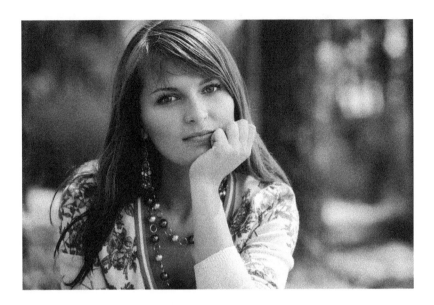

Homeopathy Treatments

Homeopathy is defined as an organic system of medicine that is based on three main ideas:

1. Like cures like

2. Minimal dosing

3. One time remedies

Alternative medicine traditionally has the least amount of "active" ingredient possible, with the concept of using one single remedy irregardless of how many symptoms are presenting. Homeopathy focuses on the least amount of treatments for better health.

There are several reasons why homeopathy is the second most popular form of medicine (after conventional medicine). The most popular reasons are:

- It is extremely natural and safe

- The results are permanent

- It is effective

- You can take most homeopathic medicines along with conventional medicine without side effects

- It is non-addictive

Homeopathy is a precise science, which is why it sometimes takes longer to find exactly the right medicine for your illness. Alternative medicine spends time asking questions about symptoms and the root cause of the illness in an effort to make a clear diagnosis for the problem, and treat it effectively.

Herbal Remedies

Nature provides many cures and treatments for ailments of all kinds. Each region has its own native plants that are used in alternative medicine.

When buying herbs for medicinal purposes, it is suggested that you use herbs from an herbal shop. Herb strength varies depending on the way in which they are grown, so until you are familiar with growing techniques for medicinal herbs, purchasing from a professional is recommended.

The Art of Alternative Medicine Made Easy

The following list provides herbal cures to common ailments:

- Acne and skin blemishes.

Wash your face and rub a clove of garlic that has been cut in half. Or, mix lavender with witch hazel at a 1:10 ratio. Tea tree oil can be substituted in place of the lavender.

- Anxiety and stress.

Lavender pure essential oil soaked onto a cotton cloth, heated, and folded into a compress. Apply to head or neck.

- Bruises and contusions.

Boil hyssop flowers and leaves into a tincture. Filter liquid, and soak a cotton compress. Apply to bruised area by applying pressure. The hyssop, heat and pressure combination will reduce the bruise.

- Burns.

Minor burns can be treated with comfrey or aloe juice. Simply rub aloe juice into burned area. Comfrey can be crushed into a fine powder, mixed with equal parts of melted beeswax, and added to vegetable oil. Simmer over low heat for 20 minutes, and then strain mixture.

- Warts.

Either use a cut piece of garlic, placed directly on the wart or, for a less odorous cure, try dandelion juice applied repeatedly throughout the day.

Herbal Teas

An age old remedy, herbal teas are used to soothe and relive pain and stress. Many teas are actually a tincture rather than a tea. A tincture is a thicker tea that is herb-dense and is infused instead of steeped.

The following list is a list of conditions and herbal tea remedies:

- Anemia.

Drink a tincture made from boiled stinging nettle leaves.

- Arthritis.

Drink a tincture of devil's claw, juniper, birch, or celery seed (not the type on your spice rack).

- Chemotherapy side effects.

Drink a tincture of Siberian ginseng root. It soothes the insides and relieves fatigue.

- Colic in babies.

Add less than 10 drops of dill and fennel tincture to their bottle.

- Constipation.

Drink a liter of rhubarb root per day.

- Cough.

Drink a tea made from garlic bulbs and ribwort leaves.

- Depression.

Drink a tincture daily made from the ground up oat plant and St. John's wart flowers.

- Fever.

Drink a hot tea made of lemon balm, yarrow, and ginger.

- Gas.

Drink a tea made of caraway, fennel, ginger, and peppermint.

- Flu symptoms.

Drink a tincture made of Echinacea, yarrow, and catnip.

Vitamins & Minerals

Taking a vitamin supplement is not a substitution for eating healthfully. However, it does serve as insurance to be certain that you are getting all of the vitamins and minerals that your body needs.

Vitamins are essential to the optimized functioning of your body. Without sufficient vitamins, for example, your blood will not clot. You need vitamins to fight colds, and boost your immune system.

It is best to take a homeopathic test to determine the vitamins that you need. This will avoid a dangerous overdose. Then you can take the vitamins you need individually, as needed, and avoid a multi-vitamin, which is chockfull of fillers.

This method will save you money, too.

Bee Therapy (aka Apitherapy)

The practice of Apitherapy is the use of bee stings, bee pollen, propolis, royal jelly, and honey to treat a variety of ailments. While there has not been extensive testing in the scientific world to validate the claims of apitherapists, history proves that the treatments provide relief.

There are five honeybee products that are used in apitherapy:

1. Venom: A practitioner will aid the patient in injecting or being stung by bees in the affected area. The venom is used to provide relief for conditions such as tendonitis, Multiple Sclerosis, and degenerative bone disease. It works because the venom is a natural anti-inflammatory which is more potent than others available to conventional medicine such as hydrocortisone. You must get tested to be certain that you are not allergic to beestings prior to exposing yourself to bee venom.

2. Pollen: A natural energy supplement that is also used as a seasonal allergy aid. It is also believed to slow down the development of wrinkles.

3. Raw Honey: A source of quick energy, raw honey is used for many cures. It can even be used as a salve on top of an open wound to avoid the spread of bacteria.

4. Royal Jelly: Is the milky white substance that the worker bees produce to feed the queen. While unsubstantiated, this substance is used as a beauty aid and is believed to help lower cholesterol.

5. Propolis: Is the glue used to keep the hives together and make repairs. Propolis is made from the sap of poplar and conifer trees. It is used to make lip balm and salves, and is considered to be an antioxidant.

Iridology

Iridology is name for the practice of determining a person's toxicity based on the color of their iris. This concept goes back to Sweden and Hungary where physicians used it to gauge disease in their patients.

For centuries, famous physicians and scientists, all the way back to the Greek physician Hippocrates; have found the people with injuries get black marks across the iris of their eye. These marks later disappear as the person's ailments heal.

In today's world, iridology is used as a preventative measure to gauge if there is a change in a person's health. It is unfortunate that iridology cannot be used to identify a specific disease.

The way in which iridology is practiced today is that the colored part of the eye (the iris) is carefully photographed using a strong camera lens. It is painless, and it takes about an hour to complete. The photos are then enlarged, and a trained professional iridologist studies it for signs of possible illness.

Even conventional doctors use the eyes as an early warning sign of bad things going on inside of the body. This study is just the more focused analysis of the iris when looking for signs of degenerative health issues.

Meditation in Healing

Meditation is a skill that is learned. Once you know how to do it properly, it can be used to greatly improve your quality of life and health.

The benefits of meditation are an increased level of energy, a more positive attitude, a better immune health, better sleep quality, and the slowing of the aging process.

To take advantage of the maximum benefit, meditate for at least 20 minutes per day prior to bedtime.

Follow these steps for meditating. First, sit down and get comfortable in a quiet room. Keep your back and neck straight, and clear your mind so that you are focusing on the present moment.

Then become aware of your breathing. Breathe in and out of your mouth, and pay attention to your stomach rising and falling.

If thoughts come into your head, acknowledge them and let the pass through your mind. Remain conscious of your breathing and relax. If your thoughts carry you away, don't get frustrated. Simply return back to focusing on your breathing.

When your time meditating is finished, become aware of your surroundings and stand up slowly.

Meditation is a wonderful way to instantly relax yourself and reenter your being. It is the perfect supplement to any treatment, both alternative and contemporary.

This deep relaxation technique will help remove stress and anxiety from life. Reduced stress can only help healing.

The Art of Alternative Medicine Made Easy
Tai Chi & Yoga

Tai Chi is a very gentle form of exercise that anyone can do. Since most people spend most of their time sitting, it is imperative that regular exercise become a part of their daily routine. Tai Chi can become that daily movement.

Exercise helps by improving circulatory function, reducing headache tension, lowering blood pressure, and eliminating chronic back and neck pain.

Tai Chi is a series of movements and stretches that anyone can do from any position, even sitting. The exercise will improve posture, stamina, and flexibility.

Movements in Tai Chi are slow and deliberate, and easy to learn. Attending a class is the best way to learn Tai Chi. Do not worry about not being in shape; Tai Chi is known to be an exercise that is done by all types of people, of all ages.

Yoga

Yoga is a great exercise activity for all types of people. It is not difficult, but you do have to want to learn about it. The main goal of yoga is to create a balanced relationship between you physical and mental health.

Yoga is a way of life that is carried throughout the day, not just while in yoga class. Yoga creates an awareness of yourself and your day to day life. This is a drastic change to many people who often live on autopilot.

You can decide how you want to use yoga, for its basic purpose of bringing together mind and body, or as more of a strenuous activity for exercise purposes.

In yoga, it is best to start out at the lowest level possible and work your way up as you develop strength and understanding. Just like most other things, it is important to know the foundational concepts before branching out into more difficult territory,

You can take instructor-led classes, or learn at home through the wide variety of DVDs.

Birkram Yoga

Birkram yoga is also known as "hot yoga", mainly because it is practiced in a space that has been heated to over 115 degrees. Hot yoga mainly focuses on stretches and balance. It also is filled with moves that create pressure in the body that blocks circulation. By going through the movements, the constant build up of pressure created by stretching are then released, providing a rush of blood through the veins. This is believed to clean them out.

There are 26 poses in hot yoga. The purpose for the hot environment in Birkram yoga is the warmth warms the body's muscles and tendons which aids in flexibility.

There are a few tips for people considering this type of yoga. First, because it is practiced in a hot room, you will sweat a lot. It is best to wear appropriate light clothing. It is also a good idea to drink plenty of water prior to your session.

The Art of Alternative Medicine Made Easy

Hatha Yoga

The main focus of Hatha yoga is breathing, meditation, and posture. The practice of this form of yoga is perfect for people that are new to it. Hatha yoga has more of a strong emphasis on the mental component of meditation, mixed in with yoga.

Karma Yoga

The Karma form of yoga pulls together the spiritual and physical worlds. The fundamentals of Karma yoga are based in the Hindu philosophy and religion. It combines two competing philosophies in the world; from the West – that life should be pleasure based, and from the East – that life should be lived for knowledge. Both theories are blended in karma.

Your karma growth is dependent on how you live your life. Bad karma comes from living your life for the purpose of money, wealth, and material possessions. Good karma comes from living your life for happiness and love.

Karma yoga helps you focus on your life as you learn about your life goals, and helps guide you in the right direction.

Neuro Linguistic Programming (NLP)

Neuro Linguistic Programming can be considered the power of positive thought and prayer. It is well documented throughout science and medicine that having a positive attitude, outlook, and having a positive support system surround you is one of the most effective alternative medicines available.

NLP is a method of programming your thoughts in order to be positive. This technique focuses on your sub-conscious and your dreams. It is imperative to truly believe that you can heal yourself for NLP to work.

How do you practice NLP? First, take a strategy that you know creates success in other areas of your life, and apply it to your healing process. You absolutely must have faith in your body's healing ability for this to work.

Muscular and Skeletal Alternative Medicine

There are numerous other alternative treatments for the skeletal and muscular systems of the body. They include:

1. Kinesiology

Professionals test the various muscles throughout the body to determine areas that are not balanced properly, and then restore balance by using a variety of techniques.

2. Rolfing

Rolfing is the use of pressure to massage the connective tissue within the body. This allows for the body to be more flexible and be aligned properly. Rolfing will provide more energy and less anxiety.

3. Massage Therapy

Massage therapy is used to break up the knotted muscles, and to retrain the muscles. It works the ligaments, tendons, and soft tissue muscles. Massage therapy increases circulation and improves breathing.

The Art of Alternative Medicine Made Easy

4. Color therapy

Color therapy uses color and light to treat ailments. Often considered a complementary treatment, color therapy is used in addition to other treatment.

There are seven colors that correspond to the wavelength centers of the body. Each color is matched with a region of the body.

5. Magnetic energy

The use of magnetic energy fields to, as magnetic therapists believe, to manipulate cells with magnetic energy. They also believe they can recharge cells. Magnetic energy can also increase blood flow that will then reduce scars on organs, provide migraine relief, and other reoccurring pain.

6. Craniosacral therapy (CST)

The craniosacral system is the membranes and fluid that envelopes the brain and spinal cord. By applying gentle pressure to the head, the rhythm of the cranioscaral system can be evaluated and in some ways manipulated. This improves the flow and function of the central nervous system. This treatment is used in alternative medicine as a preventative measure. Professional craniosacral therapy practitioners believe they can locate and release energy cysts by unblocking them and realigning the neck.

Acupuncture

In acupuncture, thin needles are inserted into the skin to draw nerve stimulation at pinpointed locations around the body. Acupuncture is a Chinese medical procedure that involves Dao – the advocate for living in balance and moderation, with ying and yang – two life elements that are opposing forces that when balanced brings good health and happiness. Acupuncture brings relief of pain, aids respiratory illnesses, and relieves headaches and ulcers, among other physical issues. It also balances the qi life force.

Reiki

Reiki is the practice of transferring healing energy from the healer's hands to the ill person. This can be done hands-on and from a distance. The healer is believed to be full of universal energy. It is thought that the practitioner can use Reiki energy to alter the frequency of the aura. Healing is achieved first physically, then emotionally, and finally spiritually.

Crystals: A Tool for Healing

Crystals have long been associated with alternative healing. A crystal is created when crystalline is formed by minerals being arranged in a precise pattern.

Quartz is the most popular crystal. The belief behind the use of crystals is that blocked energy will be released when the crystal is placed at specific points around the body.

Chapter 4- The Attributes of Herbs as Alternative Medicine

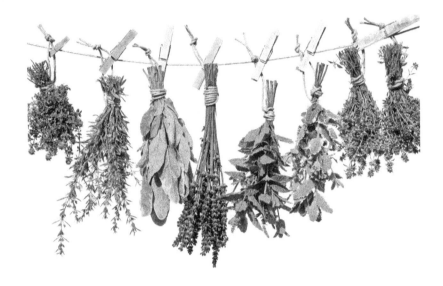

Disease isn't complicated it's really very easy and the application of good sense techniques may defeat any disease. All microbes and viruses are weak and may be defeated easily with cleaning and nutrition.

Disease is a joke if you recognize what to do and you're willing to do what it takes to heal yourself. And as they state "the truth will set you free"; and that's simply where you can, free. If you require drama and a health system that's more about disease than it is about wellness, simply go to your nearest doctor or hospital solely. If you're seeking vibrant health and a long and fruitful life you've come to the correct place for complimentary therapy.

With the increase of diseases, illnesses, and ailments sometimes turning to just medical science is not enough. Besides being costly some of the treatments can be long and stressful, further adding to the already depressive conditions.

The use of herbal healing as a form of treatment is almost considered normal in non industrialized countries. Here the traditions dictate the use of herbal healing.

Herbal healing is fast gaining popularity in the past decade. Though practiced in many ancient cultures as the first recourse to healing, it is just becoming a sought after style of healing for the modern world.

The availability of herbal healing products is no longer limited to what the older generation can prepare but is now available for all, in drug stores, supermarkets, pharmacies and other conventional outlets.

With thousands of herbs and combinations available to treat the various ailments, all it takes is a little research to find the ones that suit the needs at hand.

Though considered relatively safe because of the natural factor these herbs consists of, nevertheless is would be wise to seek the guidance of someone who is well versed in the practice of using herbs to heal, treat or control a certain condition.

As most of the herbal concoctions are fairly concentrated there may be the danger that some of the ingredients though natural may have adverse effects on the individual.

The basis of many pharmaceutical forays is in the vast possibilities of herbal healing compounds and ingredients. A lot of money and time is put into the researchers of finding and promoting the next best herbal cure for the various medical conditions the world faces today.

This is further recommended because of the little or no side effects in its consumption and also because of all the natural elements it contains when compared to chemically based and produced medications.

How to Treat Wounds with Herbs

There are lots of different herbs for different uses, made available by nature itself. Treating wounds with simple ingredients found in a household is not uncommon.

A person who prefers to treat ailments the natural way should take the time to compile a simple list of some common herbs and keep these herbs at hand to quick and easy use.

It's very handy to have some knowledge on herbs used for treating wound for children. Almost every day a child will manage to get him or herself hurt while playing, thus having these quick easy remedies available would eliminate the need to run to a medical facility often.

The aloe herb contains compounds that can reduce inflammation, swelling, and redness of wounds. This herb should be applied directly to the wound after a simple cleaning exercise is done to rid the wound of any unwanted particles. The naturally secreted gel works wonders for superficial wounds.

Calendula officinalis is another herd that can successfully treat wounds. The flavanoids and antioxidants it contain helps to speed up the healing process by increasing the blood flow to the wound. This ingredient can be applied topically and is also a popular ingredient in creams and ointments.

Slippery elm, a tree native to North America can also be used to treat wounds. Slippery elm is also found in powder form, but should be applied around the wound and not directly into an open wound.

Other more familiar herbs used to treat wounds are lavender which not only helps the healing process but also acts as a germ killing agent. Tea tree oil also disinfects while healing wounds. This particular herb works at quite a fast pace in the healing process. Echinacea, Marigold, and Myrrh are also good healing agents for wounds. All these can be applied to the wounds by simply diluting a little herbal tincture with water.

Acne Treatment with Herbs

Acne is a condition that is caused by the over production of sebum. When this happens the pores become blocked and hard plugs are formed.

This chocking eventually causes the acne condition. Other causes may include hormonal imbalances, pregnancy, menstrual periods, emotional stress, and others.

Treating the acne problem can be quite a challenge because of its reoccurring possibilities. However some advocate the use of certain herbs for better control or eradication of the acne condition.

The following are just some common suggestions of herbs used to treat acne in varying degrees.

- Tea tree oil – this treatment causes less drying and stinging after effects. Also the redness is at a minimal.

- Aloe gel – has antibacterial properties which help to kill of the germs or also stop them from contaminating other parts of the skin

- Rose water – is applied to give relief to the itching and pain

- Walnut leaf – can be used as an astringent face wash.

- Burdock root and dandelion – both these herbs contain insulin which can improve the skin condition and remove the bacteria.

- Goldenseal – helps to stop the acne from secreting any puss of other undesirable liquids.

- Calendula – promotes the healing of the tissues at a more rapid pace. It also helps to heal the scars left to some level of smoothness.

It is highly recommended that the acne condition be treated internally as well as externally. Both these areas are intertwined and treating one without the other may not produce the desired results.

When the desired results are forthcoming the conditions may end up becoming worse because now the added factor of depression and stress is added.

Acne responds to a combination of herbs used both for internal as well as external use. This combination is important to achieve long lasting results.

Ideally the herbs used for topical purposes should include tea tree oil, lavender, and calendula, while those used internally should be milk thistle and dandelion.

Chapter 5 - Take Alternative Medicine for Anxiety, Depression and Cancer

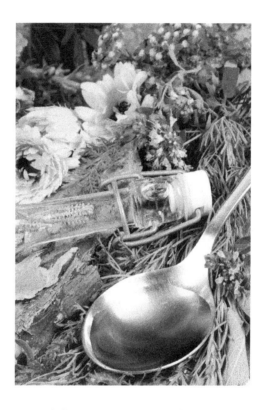

Treating anxiety and depression using herbs is a good alternative to using the conventional method of prescription drugs. This side effects from resorting to using prescription drugs and be long term, harmful and sometimes not adequately addressing the anxiety and depression issues.

By using herbal remedies it allows the person in the anxiety and depression condition to be treated through a natural way which deals with the social anxiety disorder and the body's chemical imbalance which causes the depression in the first place.

The Art of Alternative Medicine Made Easy

Of course there are some herbs that are found to be more effective than others when treating these conditions. It should be noted however that in order for these herbs to have the desired success rate or results, the diet of the individual must be well balance and healthy.

All these elements combined together will contribute to a better sense of calm and relaxed mental state.

- Magnolia bark is a powerful herbs used to treat the insomnia problem which is one of the underlying causes for depression and anxiety.

- Phellodendron bark is another fundamental herb used in ancient Chinese medicine to actually arrest the stress build up and also relief the anxiety condition. It works by regulating the cortisol which is effectively the stress hormone.

- St John wort is used to treat the depression and anxiety in only small doses. So when using this herb, prudency must be exercised.

- Valerian is regarded as the most powerful herb available to address the depression and anxiety issue. It works to positively influence the body's chemical makeup of certain elements.

- Lemon balm is also popularly referred to as the calming herb. It is mostly used for its almost sedative like inducing properties.

- Hops powder formally used primarily to treat insomnia, is now recommended for its assistance in treating depression. However at this point, it is still not conclusively proven that this herb is the only contributing factor in the success of treating depression.

Fighting Cancer

As cancer is now becoming a common and feared disease, the race is on to find a cure that is quick, easy, and accessible to everyone. Most of the current medical options available are either too costly or simply too stressful.

However as most people have no choice, they either opt not to have any treatment or decide to go through the suffering with the hope of gaining back some semblance of their previous lives.

Herbal remedies offer an alternative. Some people recommend that these herbal remedies be used alongside the current ongoing treatments and some don't.

The deciding factor would be the level of advancement the cancer stage is in. Also to be noted is the type of cancer the patient is suffering from, as different herbs work differently to address the various conditions caused by cancer.

Below are some tried and true herbs used to treat specific cancer conditions:

- Breast cancer – broccoli and green tea

- Colon cancer – broccoli

- Esophageal cancer – green tea

- General cancer – aloe vera and periwinkle

- Liver cancer – green tea

- Lung cancer – aloe vera and broccoli

- Pancreatic cancer – green tea

- Preventive cancer – broccoli, carrot, tarragon and tomato

- Prostate cancer – aloe vera, fennel and green tea

- Rectal cancer – broccoli

- Skin cancer – green tea

- Stomach cancer – aloe vera, broccoli, garlic and green tea

- Testicular cancer – periwinkle

- Cancer treatment – aloe vera, Echinacea, lantana and violet

- Cancer sores – goldenseal, lavender

There are also some herbs that help to keep the body in better shape so it then is equipped with the necessary elements to fight off the cancer cell or arrest its progressive destructive state.

Herbs like:

- Astragalus

- dong quai

- Echinacea

- shiitake

- and maitake mushrooms

All have these properties to help in the fight against cancer. However relying on these herbs alone is not advisable.

Another herb that is popular in arresting the cancer cells from its destructive nature is the mistletoe. Mistletoe preparations are commonly used to stimulate the immune system and to kill cancer cells effectively. In some extreme cases it has been noted to shrink cancer causing tumors.

Herbs For Headaches And Tension

Suffering from headaches and tension is almost part of most people's daily life. Sometimes it becomes so "normal" that is not taken seriously enough to be addressed specifically.

Instead most take the easiest solution available which is pill popping. Certainly not a long term solution, neither is it a wise thing to disregard, however using the herbal remedy alternative may be the one way of solving this condition permanently.

There are many types of herbs available to treat the annoying symptoms of headaches and tension. Some herbs are formulated to treat the conditions topically while others are meant for internal consumptions.

Herbs made into ointments and creams serve just as well and don't really cause any adverse negative effects to the individual. However, some of these ingredients can be quite strong smelling, but it's all part of inducing the comfort element to treat the conditions.

Tiger balm, peppermint oil, and nutmeg oil are just some examples of headache and tension healing herbal concoctions. Below is a list of possible herbs to choose from when addressing the headache and tension conditions:

- Feverfew – ability to prevent and stop headaches

- Ginkgo biloba – improves the circulation and decreases inflammations

- Chamomile – relaxes the body

- Peppermint – simulates the refreshing aura

- Valerian – acts as a powerful sedative

- Lemon balm and passion flower – arrest a possible attack

- Rosemary – calming effect

Besides trying all the different herbs to starve off these inconvenient and sometimes even painful conditions, keeping a healthy lifestyle and a balanced diet also helps to assist in the better state of body and mind.

Therefore when a possible attack of a headache or tension sets in, the effective use of the herbal remedy is heightened. In some cases a topical application may be adequate in addressing the condition quickly and effectively.

These kinds of applications are always a better option to choose from rather than having to consume the herbs.

Chapter 6- Alternative Medicine Affects Your Overall Wellness

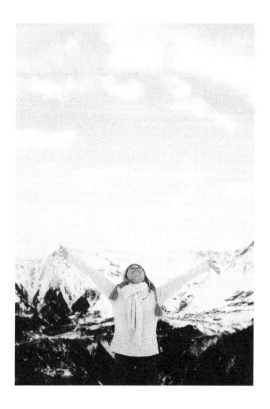

Bad eating habits and poor lifestyle practices will eventually lead to a serious level of negative elements store in the body over time. These elements also known as toxins can cause serious damage, which can and will eventually lead to illnesses, ailments, and diseases.

Addressing this critical issue is of utmost urgency, and doing it with the help of herbs is a prudent choice to make. This is because herbs are natural compounds and will not further add to any existing negative conditions.

Clean Up The Body

While some herbs are smooth others can be rough on the body, thus it is always better to start off with the gentler choice when attempting a detox session.

Psyllium is an herb derived from the seed of a fleawort plant. When in contact with liquid it expands. Psyllium is ideal for cleaning out the intestines by removing the toxins. Because of its high fiber content it also assists in "scrubbing" the digestive system effectively. However as this herb tends to absorb a lot of liquid, it is important to drink a lot of water when choosing to use this method of detox.

Aloe vera juice is also great for the digestive system as it works to kill the parasites, yeast, bacteria, and viruses. The laxative effect it helps stimulate is for detox purposes.

Cascara sagrada has long been used in ancient traditional concoctions for its detox qualities. It not only functions as an effective laxative but also helps ease constipation problems. However because this herb is rather strong, it is not advisable to use it for longer that one week.

Fennel seed is also another herb popularly used in detox exercises. Mainly used to induce bowel movements it also helps relieve gas pains and cramps in the gastrointestinal tract.

Individuals who tend to consume mainly meat and processed foods should attempt detox sessions, but it should not be done too regularly.

Breathing Better

Lung disease is popularly linked to smoking, however of late there are other factors which seem to also be linked to lung problems. The quality of air most people breathe today is really very polluted.

Some foods eaten as cooked or prepared raw also contain a lot of unwanted chemical that is the cause of lung problems too.

Numerous herbs have been known to have the necessary elements to help treat lung diseases. Asthma, lung cancer, influenza, and chronic obstructive pulmonary disease are just some of the conditions that can be treated with the use of herbal concoctions.

Licorice is an herb that may have some benefits when used to treat lung disease. Bronchitis and lung infections usually decrease of even get eradicated from using licorice regularly. It can also be used to milder conditions like inflamed throat or coughs.

Elecampane is mainly used as an antiseptic which help to kill of the existing germs and also treat the lungs and throat to prevent the reoccurrence of the infection.

It can also be used to treat irritable coughs, bronchitis, tuberculosis, silicosis, asthma, and emphysema. However as this herb can cause adverse effects like vomiting, diarrhea and stomach spasms, and a doctor should be consulted to get the right dosage.

Asian ginseng, also known as Panax ginseng may be helpful in treating lung diseases too. The ginseng is generally used to treat numerous conditions, boost the overall health and also to further support the immune system. In some cases a highly significant reduction is tumors have been noted. Ginseng can be taken as dietary supplement.

The Art of Alternative Medicine Made Easy

To provide a wider range of herbs that can be used for loosely categorized lung diseases, refer to the information given below:

- Lungs that are too dry – wild cheery bark, raw rehmannia root, glehnia root, licorice root, slippery elm bark and marshmallow root.

- Lungs that are very weak – astragalus root, cordyceps mushroom, schizandra berries, amla fruit, ginseng root, and American ginseng root.

- Simple mild lung inflammation – boswellia gum, scute root, and turmeric root.

Alternative Medicine to Keep at All Times

Using herbs to treat certain simple medical conditions have become quite common today. This eliminated the need to seek a medical practitioner every time there is a mishap, especially when there are children involved.

Mint –

There are so many uses for mint that the discovery of its uses is never ending. It's wonderful refreshing and energizing qualities is useful in pepping up teas, as a breath freshener, as an energizer, to name a few. It is also popularly used in salads and drinks.

This herb is also useful to help boost poor digestive systems and eases any gas buildups and stomach aches. Mint has antifungal properties.

Ginger –

This herb is not easy to grow but is readily available in any supermarket. It comes in either a dried form or a fresh. It is also used in many candies in its milder form.

Ginger helps in calming indigestion, painful gas buildups, other stomach discomforts, and upsets. It also helps to increase circulation. It is also a popular ingredient in Chinese style cooking.

Lemon balm –

This herb has long been used to treat anxiety and insomnia issues. Besides its antiviral and antibacterial properties it is also a great health booster and helps to shorten the duration of colds and flues in kids. In the summer time when insect bites, minor scrapes, and tummy upsets are the norm having this herb handy is an advantage.

Chamomile –

Is a favorite for treating colic, gas restlessness, and anxiety issues. It contains properties that can induce drowsiness and help calm irritable kids. It also makes for a great relaxing cup of tea.

Thyme –

This is great herb for cooking, mainly for chicken and fish. It is also great in soups and stews. Tummy cramps and gas buildups can also be treated with this herb.

Cautions

Although popularly looked upon as harmless, herbs taken without proper knowledge and supervision can have adverse and sometime serious effect on an individual. Having some knowledge about what the herb can do, how it effects in general and specifically and at what dosage is most important.

Also to be noted is that herbs should not be taken in place of ongoing medical treatments without the approval of the medical practitioner involved.

Some herbs when taken with other conventional medication can cause the medication to lose its usefulness and this may be detrimental to the individual who really needs the medically prescribed medication. Herbs can also alter the makeup of some medication when ingested along with it. Thus instead of being an added value it becomes a problem instead. Therefore again medical advice should be sought before considering the line of treatment even if it is only a supplementary element.

Upon understanding and getting the approval from a medical practitioner, the dosage to take is also a very important item to consider. As the herb maybe new to the body system, taking it in large doses or too frequently may shock the system and at worse cause a complete shutdown. In some extreme cases death has been the result of ingesting unfamiliar herbs.

People who are easily influences should be especially weary and careful as to what herbs they buy. Many unscrupulous vendors will promote the positive side of their herbal products without ever disclosing the possible negative findings. In some cases the negative findings are played down so as not to frighten a potential customer off.

Sometimes instead of seeking medical advice immediately upon discovering an illness, ailment, or disease, the choice is made to embark upon trying to treat the condition with using herbs. This may cause the individual to lose precious time in arresting the negative condition or even worse cause further damage.

The healing by plants is the most popular and oldest therapy for healing on the globe. The info regarding herbal nutrition has been transplanted from one generation to other since the very start.

Due to the development of the process of synthetic medicine or drug making, the utilization of herbs got to be a movement of past. All the same, there's a sudden increase in the practice of utilization of herbs for treatment of ill health which is inexpensive, secure and natural.

The key aim of utilizing herbal remedies is to expand the procedure of natural healing inside body by rebalancing and cleansing. A few herbals hold antiviral and antibacterial qualities like synthetic medicines and drugs. The advantages of the technique of herbal healing are that it brings the body back to normal state without presenting a lot of side effects.

The right combination of herbs may be used to heal and tone up body or tainted tissues.

Herbs may be utilized to focus, heal, control or tone any part of body if they're recommended or combined in suitable manner. Herbs ought to be consumed with proper counsel of a practitioner.

Chapter 7 - Herbal Teas Recipes as Alternative Medicine

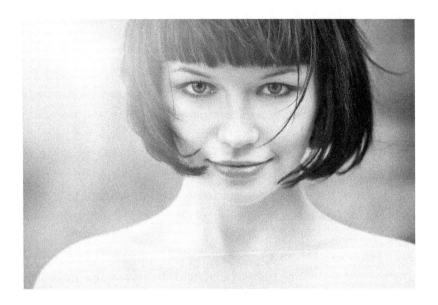

There are so many ways that our immune systems can be overwhelmed ... it's in our air, our water, our food, our workplace, our stress. This blend of organic and wild herbs is not only helpful but comforting, strengthening and tasty.

1 part red clover blossoms 1 part nettle leaves

1 part pau d'Arco

1 part alfalfa & sage leaves 1 part St.Johns wort tops

1 part ginger root

Place all herbs in a tea ball or bag, put in your nicest or most favorite cup or mug, and cover with boiling water. Steep for 10 minutes.

Remove tea ball or bag, and add sugar, honey, sweetener, milk, cream or whatever, to taste.

ADD/ADHD Remetea

Teaspoon Hops

1 Teaspoon Gotu Kola

Bring 1 1/2 cups of water to a boil. Place the herbs inside, place lid on tightly and let it steep for 5 minutes. Drink twice a day.

After Dinner Carminative Tea

1 cup water

1 tablespoon fennel seeds

Bring the water and fennel seeds to a boil with the lid on the pan and let sit for 15 minutes and enjoy this calming cup of tea. Fennel is a wonderful herb for digestion and can help your body increase its ability to digest a big meal or a meal with lots of fat.

Allergy Season Blend

Cool minty, citrus flavor to assist you with the discomfort associated with allergy season.

1 part nettle

1 part peppermint

1 part spearmint 1 part yerba santa 1 part eyebright

1 pat lemongrass leaves 1 part calendula

The Art of Alternative Medicine Made Easy

1 part red clover

1 part lavender flowers 1 part fennel seeds

a pinch of stevia

Place all herbs in a tea ball or bag, put in your nicest or most favorite cup or mug, and cover with boiling water. Steep for 10 minutes.

Remove tea ball or bag, and add sugar, honey, sweetener, milk, cream or whatever, to taste.

Aphrodite Blend Tea

A sensuous, aromatic blend with just the right tint of zest for your palate, and sure to kindle flames! A delicate, but dashing combination makes this one of your most enjoyable cups of tea.

1 part Damiana leaves 1 part rose petals

1 part peppermint leaves 1 part muira puama

1 part gingko leaves 1 part orange peel

1 part cinnamon bark chips pinch of stevia.

Place all herbs in a tea ball or bag, put in your nicest or most favorite cup or mug, and cover with boiling water. Steep for 10 minutes.

Remove tea ball or bag, and add sugar, honey, sweetener, milk, cream or whatever, to taste.

Bladder Infections Tea

1 ½ oz dried Goldenrod 1/4 oz Juniper Berries*

3/4 oz chopped Dandelion root 3/4 oz chopped Rose Hips

Pour 1 cup boiling water over 2 tsp of mixture. Steep 10 minutes & strain.

can become toxic, so only drink 2 cups of this mixture daily for no more than 3 days

Blood Builder Tea

1 tsp Rose Hips-crushed 1 Tsp Butcher's Broom 1 Tsp Yellow Dock

Bring 31/2 cups of water to a boil. Remove water from heat and add herbs. Place a tight lid on the pot. Let the mixture steep for five to ten minutes. Drink one cup three times daily. Yields three cups.

Blossoms of Health Tea

Beautiful to look at, nectar to taste and good for you. A popular tea. Spirited, uplifting and energizing.

1 part ginkgo leaves 1 part red clover tops 1 part nettle leaves

1 part meadowsweet leaves 1 part calendula

2 parts chamomile

2 parts lavender flowers 1 part gotu kola leaves a pinch of stevia.

Place all herbs in a tea ball or bag, put in your nicest or most favorite cup or mug, and cover with boiling water. Steep for 10 minutes.

Remove tea ball or bag, and add sugar, honey, sweetener, milk, cream or whatever, to taste.

Blues Tea

1 part Nettle leaves,

1 part St Johns wort tops 2 parts spearmint

1 part damiana leaves 1 part kava kava root

a tiny pinch of stevia to taste

Place all herbs in a tea ball or bag, put in your nicest or most favorite cup or mug, and cover with boiling water. Steep for 10 minutes.

Remove tea ball or bag, and add sugar, honey, sweetener, milk, cream or whatever, to taste.

Breast Health Tea

2 parts calendula 2 parts red clover 1 part cleavers

1 part lady's mantle

Spearmint or peppermint (optional; for flavor)

Prepare as an infusion, using 1 ounce of herbs per quart of water, and letting steep overnight. Drink 3 to 4 cups daily.

Bronchial Congestion Tea

1 ½ oz Aniseed

1 oz Calendula flowers 3/4 oz Marshmallow root 1/3 oz Licorice root

Crush aniseeds and add to herbs. Pour 1 cup boiling water over 1 tsp mixture; cover & steep 10 minutes.

Calming Tea 1

1 oz Lemon balm

1 oz Chamomile flowers

½ oz St John's Wort

Steep 2 tbs of mixture in 1 cup boiled water. Cover 10 minutes; strain.

Calming Tea 2

1 Part Sage

1 Part Thyme

1 Part Marjorham

1 Part Chamomile

Blend ingredients in a tea ball and put in a mug of hot water

The Art of Alternative Medicine Made Easy

Colds and Flu Tea

1 oz Blackberry leaves 1 oz Elder flowers

1 oz Linden flowers

1 oz Peppermint leaves

Pour 1 cup boiling water over 2 tbs mixture. Cover & steep 10 minutes; strain.

Colds and Hoarseness Tea

2 oz Malva flowers

1 ½ oz Mullein flowers

Use 2 tbs of mixture per 1 cup hot water. Steep 10 minutes; strain. Drink only 2 - 3 cups per day for just a few days.

Winter Tea

Boneset Echinacea Peppermint

Just use equal parts of each, or pre-made tea bags...3 bags, 1 of boneset,1 of echinacea, and 1 of peppermint.

The echinacea works as an immune system builder, the boneset is great for congestion, aches and fever (the classic flu symptoms), and the peppermint aids with any stomach complaints due to drainage from the sinuses, and just works as a great overall "feel-good".

Coughing Fits Tea

1 1/3 oz. St. John's Wort 2/3 oz. Thyme

2/3 oz. Linden Flowers

Use 1 tsp. of the herb mixture per cup of boiling water to soothe irritations of the upper respiratory tract that cause coughing. Steep for 5-10 min., strain, sweeten if necessary. This tea has proved helpful with bronchitis and whooping cough.

Crone Root Tea

For menopause and beginning a new cycle of life. 2 tablespoons wild yam

2 tablespoons licorice

3 tablespoons sarsaparilla 1 tablespoon chaste berry 1 tablespoon ginger

1 tablespoon false unicorn root 2 tablespoons sage

1 tablespoon cinnamon

½ tablespoon black cohash

Detoxification Tea

1 tsp Green Tea leaves

Simmer 1 cup water & pour over leaves. Cover & let stand 4 minutes.

The Art of Alternative Medicine Made Easy

Dream Tea

2 parts Rose

1 part Mugwort

1 part Peppermint

1 part Jasmine

1/2 part Cinnamon Drink to cause dreams.

Combine all ingredients thoroughly, fill tea diffuser @ 1 tsp. per cup of boiling water and as it steeps say;

Dual Purpose Tea

Do not drink more than 2 cups a day.

2 teaspoons dried German Chamomile flowers 1 cup boiling water

Steep the flowers in the boiling water, covered, for 15 minutes. Strain, then slowly sip the infusion to relieve nausea, stomach upset, and lessen menstrual cramps.

Echinacea & Roots Tea

A tasty way to help strengthen and support your natural resistance. A very popular tea.

1 partechinacea purpurea root 1 part pau d'arco

1 part dandelion root (raw and roasted) 1 part sarsaparilla bark

1 part cinnamon barks 1 part ginger root

1 part burdock roots 1 part sassafras bark a pinch of stevia

Place all herbs in a tea ball or bag, put in your nicest or most favorite cup or mug, and cover with boiling water. Steep for 10 minutes.

Remove tea ball or bag, and add sugar, honey, sweetener, milk, cream or whatever, to taste.

Evening Repose Tea

When the sun sets over the hill and the new moon dips her silver softness, savor the tranquility in our evening repose blend. It's a perfect toast to the rising moon. A robust flavor of flowers and mint.

1 part roses

1 part lavender flowers

1 part lemon verbena leaves 1 part chamomile flowers

1 part each peppermint & spearmint leaves 1 part blue malva flowers pinch of stevia

Place all herbs in a tea ball or bag, put in your nicest or most favorite cup or mug, and cover with boiling water. Steep for 10 minutes.

Remove tea ball or bag, and add sugar, honey, sweetener, milk, cream or whatever, to taste.

The Art of Alternative Medicine Made Easy
Fever Reducer Tea

2 tsp dried Catnip 1 tsp dry Vervain

Pour 2 cups boiling water over herbs. Steep 10 minutes & strain.

Flashes Blend Tea

Brew up a pot and sip when needed. 1 part sage

1 part motherwort

1 part dandelion

1 part chickweed & violet leaves

1 part each elder flowers & oatstraw

Place all herbs in a tea ball or bag, put in your nicest or most favorite cup or mug, and cover with boiling water. Steep for 10 minutes.

Remove tea ball or bag, and add sugar, honey, sweetener, milk, cream or whatever, to taste.

Flu-away

2 medium cloves of freshly crushed garlic 1 cup of very warm water

1 teaspoon of honey

1 teaspoon of lemon juice Stir and drink.

Fluid Retention Tea

1 oz Dandelion root

1 oz Dandelion leaves 2/3 oz Nettle leaves

2/3 oz Spearmint leaves

Steep mixture in 1 cup of water for 10 minutes.

Tea for menstrual problems, fertility and childbirth.

3 tablespoons sassafras bark 2 tablespoons dandelion root 1 tablespoon ginger root

½ tablespoon cinnamon 1 tablespoon licorice root

½ tablespoon orange peel 1 tablespoon pau d'arco

¼ tablespoon dong quai root 1 tablespoon chaste berry

1 tablespoon wild yam

Forests Tea(formerly Lung Blend)

1 part echinacea purpurea 1 part elecampane

1 part ginger

1 part each pleurisy & licorice roots 1 part white oak bark

1 part cinnamon bark

1 part each orange peel and fennel seeds

The Art of Alternative Medicine Made Easy

Place all herbs in a tea ball or bag, put in your nicest or most favorite cup or mug, and cover with boiling water. Steep for 10 minutes.

Remove tea ball or bag, and add sugar, honey, sweetener, milk, cream or whatever, to taste.

Happy Man Tea Blend

1 part Siberian ginseng 1 part dandelion root

1 part nettle

1 part each marshmallow & burdock roots

1 part each hawthorn & saw palmetto berries 1 part fennel seeds

1 part wildoats a pinch of stevia

Place all herbs in a tea ball or bag, put in your nicest or most favorite cup or mug, and cover with boiling water. Steep for 10 minutes.

Remove tea ball or bag, and add sugar, honey, sweetener, milk, cream or whatever, to taste.

Climb into bed and enjoy!

Happy Tummy Tea

Put a smile on your face with this soothing and yummy tea. 1 part catnip

1 part spearmint & lemongrass leaves 1 part calendula flowers

1 part skullcap

1 part rosemary & sage leaves 1 part fennel seeds

Place all herbs in a tea ball or bag, put in your nicest or most favorite cup or mug, and cover with boiling water. Steep for 10 minutes.

Remove tea ball or bag, and add sugar, honey, sweetener, milk, cream or whatever, to taste.

Headache Tea

Lavender Chamomile Rosemary Mint

Put a pinch of each herb in a coffee filter and place in your coffee maker. Wait a half hour before drinking this mix, this should make you tired so you can sleep your headache away.

Healing Ginger tea

2 cups of water

4 tablespoons freshly grated ginger root

Place in pan with a lid on, bring to a boil, and turn off the heat and let sit for two hours. Re-heat the tea, strain the herb from the tea and drink.

Insomnia Tea

1 ½ oz dried Vervain leaves 1 oz Chamomile

½ oz Spearmint

The Art of Alternative Medicine Made Easy

Mix all and add to 1 cup boiling water. Steep 8 minutes; strain.

Less Stress Tea

Relieves stress, relaxes low back and neck areas. 1 part chamomile

1 part mint

1 part calendula flowers

Place all herbs in a tea ball or bag, put in your nicest or most favorite cup or mug, and cover with boiling water. Steep for 10 minutes.

Remove tea ball or bag, and add sugar, honey, sweetener, milk, cream or whatever, to taste.

Mellow Mood Tea

This tea is made with the most palatable of the calming herbs. Blended together, they'll defuse stress and anxiety and promote sound sleep.

WHAT YOU NEED

1 teaspoon chamomile flowers 1 teaspoon lavender spikes

1 teaspoon kava leaves

1 teaspoon lemon balm leaves 1 teaspoon marjoram

1 spray valerian flowers 1 quart water

WHAT TO DO

In a large saucepan, steep the chamomile, lavender, kava, lemon balm, marjoram, and valerian to taste in the freshly boiled water. Strain out the plant material. Drink the tea hot or cool as often as needed, refrigerating any left over for later use.

CAUTION: Chamomile is in the rag weed family, and many are allergic to herbs.

Memory Zest Blend

A mentally refreshing beverage, to help give you feelings of clarity and precision.

1 part ginkgo

1 part gotu kola and peppermint leaves 1 part red clover tops

1 part rosemary leaves 1 part ginger root

a pinch of stevia.

Place all herbs in a tea ball or bag, put in your nicest or most favorite cup or mug, and cover with boiling water. Steep for 10 minutes.

Remove tea ball or bag, and add sugar, honey, sweetener, milk, cream or whatever, to taste.

Migraine Tea

1 2/3 oz dried St John's Wort 1 oz Valerian

1 oz Linden flowers 1/4 oz Juniper berries

The Art of Alternative Medicine Made Easy

Use 1 tsp of mixture per 1 cup boiling water. Steep 10 minutes & strain.

Moon Ease Tea

For that time of the month. 2 parts crampbark

1 part chaste tree berries

1 part each spearmint & skullcap leaves 1 part marshmallow root

1 part passionflower herb 1 part ginger root

Procedure

Place all herbs in a tea ball or bag, put in your nicest or most favorite cup or mug, and cover with boiling water. Steep for 10 minutes.

Remove tea ball or bag, and add sugar, honey, sweetener, milk, cream or whatever, to taste.

My Nerves Are Shot Tea!

Uses:

Sleeplessness and Insomnia Job-related stress

Panic attacks Ingredients:

2 parts Chamomile

1 part Jasmine

1 part Hops

1 part Lavender

1 part Yerba Santa 1 part Gota Kola

1 part St. John's Wort Preparation:

Place all herbs in a tea ball or bag, put in your nicest or most favorite cup or mug, and cover with boiling water. Steep for 10 minutes.

Remove tea ball or bag, and add sugar, honey, sweetener, milk, cream or whatever, to taste.

Natural Concentration Tea

Helps you to become more creative in designing a more natural environment in your home.

1 part Celendula

1 part mint,

1 part sage (flowers only) 1 part yarrow leaves

Place all herbs in a tea ball or bag, put in your nicest or most favorite cup or mug, and cover with boiling water. Steep for 10 minutes.

Remove tea ball or bag, and add sugar, honey, sweetener, milk, cream or whatever, to taste.

Nausea Tea

½ tsp dried Ginger root

The Art of Alternative Medicine Made Easy

½ tsp Clove blossoms

1 tsp Chamomile flowers

Pour 1 cup boiling water over herbs. Steep 10 minutes, strain & let cool.

Nervous Stomach Tea

2 tsp Angelica root

2 tsp Lemon Balm leaves

½ tsp Fennel seed

Bring Angelica root to a simmer in 4 cups water. Turn off heat, add lemon balm & lemon; steep 10 minutes & strain.

Nervous Tension Tea

1 1/3 oz. St. John's Wort 1 oz. Lemon Balm Leaves 1 oz. Valerian

Use 1 tsp of the herb mixture per cup of boiling water. Steep for 10 min., strain, sweeten if necessary. Drink a cup before going to bed each night for several weeks to calm nerves, lift depression, and help you fall asleep more easily.

"No-Sweat" Tea

4 cups boiling water 1 tsp. dried hops

1 tsp. stinging nettle

1 tsp. fresh cut rose petals

1 tsp. dried strawberry leaves 1 tsp. fresh walnut leaves

3 tbsp of dried sage leaves

Reduces perspiration within 2 hours of use with its effects lasting several days:

Combine all ingredients, cover and steep for an hour. Strain and sweeten with honey if desired.

Nursing Mother's Tea

1 teaspoon crushed Fennel seeds 1 cup boiling water

Mix the seeds with the boiling water. Cover and steep for 10 minutes. Strain, and sip the infusion. Drinking a tea made with fennel helps to promote the secretion of breast milk in nursing mothers.

Pinkeye tea recipe

Fill a tea ball with equal parts chamomile(antiseptic),borag (alleviated inflammation and redness),eyebright(excellent for conjunctivitis any other eye complaints) and elderflowers(beneficial for tired eyes). pour on 2 1/2 cups boiling hot(fresh from the kettle)water allow to steep until cooled. add 5 drops witch-hazel extract(coolant and antiseptic) and stir. wash eye(outside) gently with infusion and put one drop of infusion in eye as needed or desired. also can be used by soaking a cloth in the infusion and putting over the eye until you eye feels better. if your using this for a child leave out the witch-hazel. this is good for anything where your eyes are painful inflamed and red.

The Art of Alternative Medicine Made Easy

Pleasant Dreams

1 cup mugwort

1/2 cup rose petals 1/2 cup chamomile

1/3 cup lavender flowers 1/3 cup catnip

2 tbsp mint

Quiet Child Tea

Good for anytime of the day or right before bedtime. 1 part raspberry leaves

1 part catnip

1 part each spearmint & skullcap leaves 1 part calendula flowers

a pinch of stevia

Place all herbs in a tea ball or bag, put in your nicest or most favorite cup or mug, and cover with boiling water. Steep for 10 minutes.

Remove tea ball or bag, and add sugar, honey, sweetener, milk, cream or whatever, to taste.

Quiet Time Tea

1 part oregano

2 parts Chamomile 1 part lemon balm 1 part lemon thyme

Place all herbs in a tea ball or bag, put in your nicest or most favorite cup or mug, and cover with boiling water. Steep for 10 minutes.

Remove tea ball or bag, and add sugar, honey, sweetener, milk, cream or whatever, to taste.

Rejuvenation Tea

Etheric cleanser of old, stale thoughts and patterns of behavior for new beginnings and awakening.

1 part rose hips

1 part calendula flowers

1 part gallum (cleavers) flowers 1 part borage flowers

1 part nettles leaves

Place all herbs in a tea ball or bag, put in your nicest or most favorite cup or mug, and cover with boiling water. Steep for 10 minutes.

Remove tea ball or bag, and add sugar, honey, sweetener, milk, cream or whatever, to taste.

Relaxation Tea

2 parts chamomile 1 part lemon balm 1 part lemon peel 1 part thyme

The Art of Alternative Medicine Made Easy

Place all herbs in a tea ball or bag, put in your nicest or most favorite cup or mug, and cover with boiling water. Steep for 10 minutes.

Remove tea ball or bag, and add sugar, honey, sweetener, milk, cream or whatever, to taste.

Sleep Tea Recipe

2 tbls. Hops

1 tsp. Lavender

1 tsp. Rosemary

1 tsp. Thyme

1 tsp. Mugwort

1 tsp. Sage

1 Pinch of Valerian Root

Take a teaspoon of the mixture and pour into 1 cup of hot water. Let sit for 3 minutes then strain. Store the unused portion.

Soothing Tea

1 part mint

1 part hyssop

1 part oregano

1 part parsley

1 part lemon balm

Place all herbs in a tea ball or bag, put in your nicest or most favorite cup or mug, and cover with boiling water. Steep for 10 minutes.

Remove tea ball or bag, and add sugar, honey, sweetener, milk, cream or whatever, to taste.

Spiced Relief

1 teaspoon anise seeds, crushed or ground 2-3 cinnamon sticks

1 inch of ginger, sliced

1-2 teaspoons dried loose Echinacea

Combine spices and Echinacea in a pot with three cups of water. Bring to a boil and then simmer for 15-20 minutes to make a decoction. Strain into a mug and add honey to taste. This is a multi-function tea. Anise acts as an expectorant, ginger soothes the cough, and cinnamon has anti-bacterial properties.

Tea For Health

1 tablespoon China black tea 2 teaspoon fennel

1 teaspoon mint

2 teaspoon rose hips

1 teaspoon elder flower 2 teaspoon hops

1 teaspoon mullein

The Art of Alternative Medicine Made Easy

Tea for Nervousness

1 ½ oz Peppermint leaves 1 ½ oz Lemon Balm leaves

Use 1 tsp of mixture per 1 cup boiling water. Steep 10 minutes & strain.

Tummy Tea

A wonderful tea blend to enjoy after a big meal or hectic day. 1 cup dried peppermint (or other)

1 tbsp dried rosemary 1 tsp dried sage

Crush ingredients and mix well. Store in an airtight container. Steep 1 heaping tsp in a cup of boiling water for 1 minute. Sweeten with honey.

Upset Stomach Tea

8 oz Peppermint leaves 8 oz Lemon Balm leaves 8 oz Fennel seeds

Use 1 tsp of mixture per 1 cup boiling water. Steep 10 minutes; strain.

Urinary Infection Tea

1 teaspoon uva ursi

½ teaspoon each corn silk, cramp bark, marshmallow root and rose hips

1 quart water

Simmer herbs in water for a couple of minutes, then steep them for 20 minutes. Strain herbs. Drink 2 to 4 cups daily. To make sure the infection is gone, continue taking the herbs for 2 days after the symptoms disappear.

Winter Tea

Boneset Echinacea Peppermint

Just use equal parts of each, or pre-made tea bags...3 bags, one of boneset, 1 of echinacea, and 1 of peppermint.

Wise Woman Tea

A wonderful menopause tea. Gently calms, cools and balances. 1 part motherwort

1 part sage

1 part nettle leaves

1 part each lemon balm & mugwort leaves 1 part chaste tree berries

1 part horsetail

Place all herbs in a tea ball or bag, put in your nicest or most favorite cup or mug, and cover with boiling water. Steep for 10 minutes.

Remove tea ball or bag, and add sugar, honey, sweetener, milk, cream or whatever, to taste.

Beauty From the Inside out!

The Art of Alternative Medicine Made Easy

Honey bush tea is a pleasant way to keep the body well hydrated with fluids This herbal tea has many health benefits! Honey bush has nearly the same properties as Rooibos. It is caffeine free low in tannin, and very rich in antioxidants. It contains no additives, preservatives or colorants.

The mineral found in Honey bush are Potassium, Calcium, Magnesium, Sodium, Copper, Zinc, manganese Iron and fluoride. According to ongoing research Honey bush also contains Isoflavones & Coumestans, Xanthones, Flavones, all known to promote good health and are also known to help prevent certain cancers.

Honey bush has anti-spasmodic properties which mean those with weak digestion can easily enjoy this tea. It has been a treatment for colic in babies .It also helps to relieve insomnia.

Tea - Patti's Pain Killer

The herbs you can choose from are as follows: Lady´s Mantle (herb)

Raspberry Leaf (herb) Yarrow (herb)

Chaste Tree Berry

Fennel Seed (for the stomach) Peppermint (for the stomach) Valerian (for the stomach)

Use(1) part each (choose a total of five including one for the stomach) and steep like a tea.

Stress-Reducing Rest

1/2 cup sweet hops 1/2 cup mugwort

1/8 cup sweet marjoram

All the following recipes have the same measurements. Unless otherwise stated, they were brewed in a coffee maker or tea brewer.

Measurements: 1 tablespoon of each type of herb 1 tablespoon of honey to sweeten the tea

Sore throat

Licorice root Slippery Elm Peppermint

The Common Cold

1 1/2 tablespoons of Licorice root already brewed in a pot enough for two cups.

Elderberry tea bag Chamomile

Steep the tea bag in the Licorice Root infusion and add in the Chamomile. This can be done in the coffee maker, but the Licorice brew must be cool enough to be cycled through the machine.

Stomach ache

(nausea)

Must be done in a pot on the stove.

I pod of Star Anise per cup Chamomile (bag or tea ball)

Fever buster Tea

Catnip

The Art of Alternative Medicine Made Easy

White Oak bark Chamomile

Must be ingested as hot as the person can take it. Chamomile can be substituted for any other fragrant herb. It is added in only for taste.

Dry, raspy cough

Licorice Root Slippery Elm Mullein Catnip Chamomile Honey

Lemon 1 wedge

Aches and Pains Tea

1 Tablespoon White Willow Bark 1 Tablespoon Catnip

Put in a tea ball and steep in boiling hot water for five minutes. Drink as hot as you can stand it, then lie down for a nap.

Blood Builder Tea

1 tsp Rose Hips-crushed 1 Tsp Butcher's Broom 1 Tsp Yellow Dock

Bring 3 1/2 cups of water to a boil. Remove water from heat and add herbs. Place a tight lid on the pot. Let the mixture steep for five to ten minutes. Drink one cup three times daily. Yields three cups.

Constipation Tea

1/2 teaspoon Cascara Sagrada 1 teaspoon Chamomile

Take in one dose before bedtime. One coffee cup full should do it.

Cramp Tea

1 teaspoon Cramp Bark

1 teaspoon Red Raspberry Leaves 1 teaspoon Dong Quai

Take this tea in coffee cup full glasses. This makes enough for two cups. The tea is only good for six hours.

Detox Tea

1 Teaspoon Pau D'Arco (Taheebo) 1 Teaspoon Cascara Sagrada

1 Teaspoon Echinacea

Bring 1 1/2 cups water to a boil. Place herbs into the water, cover tightly and let steep for five minutes. I cup two times a day should help. If bowels are loose, dilute combination in 2 to 2 1/2 cups water.

Dry Congestion Tea

(For thick congestion and irritated mucous membranes.)

2 parts Eyebright

1 part Catnip

2 parts Thyme

1 part Goldenrod

Steep 1-1/2 to 2 tsp in a larger cup, such as a coffee mug, for 10 minutes. You will likely need lemon or honey, as this remedy is rather bitter. Very soothing. Try to stay warm while drinking, and for a time afterwards.

**If you experience any discomfort or unpleasant effects while drinking this tea, discontinue use. All herbs listed above are generally safe, though precautions should always be taken when using any type of medicine.*

During cold or sinus season Tea

1 small handful (about 1/4 cup) dried thyme

1 small handful (about 1/4 cup) dried feverfew flowers 1 large handful (about 3/4 cup) dried peppermint leaves 1 Tablespoon dried and rubbed or crushed sage

End of Your Rope Tea

1 Tablespoon Chamomile

1 Tablespoon Peppermint

Put in a tea ball and steep in boiling hot water for five minutes.

Epilepsy Combination

1 tsp Valerian

1 tsp Skullcap

1 tsp Hops

Bring water to a boil and add herbs. Cover pot with lid and let steep for 5 minutes..

Tea For Digestive Problems

1oz. chamomile 2/3 oz. peppermint

1 oz. caraway seeds 2/3 oz. angelica

Use 1 tsp of the mixture per cup of hot water. Steep the mixture 10 min. and strain.

This tea soothes the gastrointestinal tract and stimulates digestive activity, making it useful for stomachaches or a too-full feeling

Heartburn Tea

1 tablespoon Chamomile 1 table spoon Peppermint 2 pods Star Anise

Boil pods for 5 minutes and steep the chamomile and peppermint in the Anise tea. Drink one cup every hour for two hours before bedtime.

Hops Sleep Blend

2 ounces Hops, dried

2 ounces of chamomile, dried

1/2 ounce Eucalyptus leaves, dried 1 ounce Lemon Balm

1 ounce Orris Root powder

3 drops Lemon Balm essential oil

The Art of Alternative Medicine Made Easy

Memory Minder Tea

1 tsp Gingko Biloba 1 tsp Panax Ginseng 1 tsp Peppermint

Bring two cups of water to a boil. Add herbs and place a tight lid over the pot for five to ten minutes. Take one cup in the morning and one cup around mid-day.

Stop that Cough Tea

1 tablespoon Slippery Elm 1 tablespoon Mullein

1 tablespoon Catnip

1 tablespoon Licorice root bark

Boil the bark first in two cups worth of water for 10 minutes. Place the rest of the herbs in a coffee filter and place the filter in a strainer. Strain the Licorice tea through the strainer into a mug and drink.

Honey and lemon can be added.

Super Relaxer Tea

1 part (1 teaspoon) valerian root (dried)

1 part (1 teaspoon) Chamomile flowers (dried)

In a Teapot pour in 2 mug full of hot water (not boiling) steep for 5 mins. Strain or remove tea bags.

Add honey if desired. This is great at night before bed

Adam Potts

Tranquility Tea

Mix:

2 parts Red Clover blossoms 2 parts Rose Hips

1 part German Chamomile flowers 1 part Peppermint leaves

Very Odd Cure for Bad Breath

Drink tea.

Researchers from the College of Dentistry at the University of Illinois at Chicago say compounds in tea can slow the growth of bacteria in our mouths, which is the primary cause of bad breath. The magic ingredients are antioxidants called polyphenols, and they are found in both green and black teas.

It's the bacteria that live on the back surface of the tongue and in the deep pockets between the gums and teeth that make our breath smell bad. The bacteria "make horrible, smelly stuff," lead study author Christine D. Wu explained to Reuters in an interview. "That's why we get bad breath."

Wu and her colleagues showed in earlier studies that black tea can slow dental plaque formation and help your toothpaste work more effectively. Her latest laboratory experiments have shown that tea's polyphenols not only inhibit three species of bacteria that cause halitosis, but also stop an enzyme that causes the formation of hydrogen sulfide--the ultimate culprit for rotten breath.

But here's the catch: Tea won't sweeten your breath. So don't throw out the mouthwash just yet. "All we can say is that a cup of tea will produce more than enough of these active materials to affect the bacteria," she said. "Remember, this is a lab study. In the mouth, bacteria are protected by all sorts of things."

Baby Sleep Tea

1 tsp hops

1 tsp Chamomile

Place 4 cups of water into a glass or porcelain pot and bring to a boil. Take the pot of the heat and add the herbals. Put a tight lid on the pot and let it steep for five minutes. Strain out herbals.

Place in four ounce glass bottle after it is cool enough for baby and let them drink it.

Depression Tamer Tea

1 tsp St John's Wort 1 tsp Gingko Biloba

Place 1 cup of water into a glass or porcelain pot and bring to a boil. Take the pot of the heat and add the herbals. Put a tight lid on the pot and let it steep for five minutes. Strain out herbals. Place in a cup and sweeten with honey of desired.

About The Author

Adam Potts suffered depression and anxiety when her mother passed away. He was really hurt knowing that the one person who raised him and loved him has to leave him. But Adam was not alone. He still has friends and relatives to help him and still will love him. Realizing these blessings that he had taken for granted before, he knew that he needs to help himself as well. Then, he discovered the calming effects of teas.

Adam is now a certified holistic instructor and a fitness buff. He wants to inspire and help others in whatever challenges that they may encounter.

www.ingramcontent.com/pod-product-compliance
Lightning Source LLC
LaVergne TN
LVHW012154080325
805498LV00009B/652